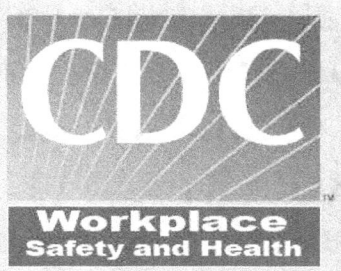

Workplace
Safety and Health

Noise and Lead Exposures at an Outdoor Firing Range – California

Lilia Chen, MS, CIH
Scott E. Brueck, MS, CIH

Health Hazard Evaluation Report
HETA 2011-0069-3140
September 2011

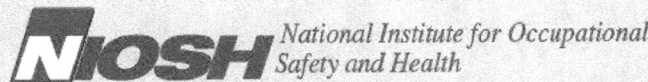

DEPARTMENT OF HEALTH AND HUMAN SERVICES
Centers for Disease Control and Prevention
National Institute for Occupational Safety and Health

The employer shall post a copy of this report for a period of 30 calendar days at or near the workplace(s) of affected employees. The employer shall take steps to insure that the posted determinations are not altered, defaced, or covered by other material during such period. [37 FR 23640, November 7, 1972, as amended at 45 FR 2653, January 14, 1980].

CONTENTS

ABBREVIATIONS

μg/100 cm^2	Micrograms per 100 square centimeters
μg/dL	Micrograms per deciliter
μg/m^3	Micrograms per cubic meter
AIHA	American Industrial Hygiene Association
ACGIH®	American Conference of Governmental Industrial Hygienists
AL	Action level
BLL	Blood lead level
CFR	Code of Federal Regulations
dB	Decibel
dBA	Decibel, A-scale
dBC	Decibel, C-scale
Hz	Hertz
m^3	Cubic meter
mg/m^3	Milligrams per cubic meter
MDC	Minimum detectable concentration
MQC	Minimum quantifiable concentration
min	Minute
MSDS	Material safety data sheet
NAICS	North American Industry Classification System
NIHL	Noise-induced hearing loss
NIOSH	National Institute for Occupational Safety and Health
NRR	Noise reduction rating
OEL	Occupational exposure limit
OSHA	Occupational Safety and Health Administration
PBZ	Personal breathing zone
PEL	Permissible exposure limit
PPE	Personal protective equipment
REL	Recommended exposure limit
SLM	Sound level meter
TLV®	Threshold limit value
TWA	Time-weighted average
WEEL™	Workplace environmental exposure level

The National Institute for Occupational Safety and Health (NIOSH) received a technical assistance request from a federal government agency in California. Although no health symptoms or hearing loss were reported, the requestor was concerned about exposures to noise and lead among firing range instructors at an outdoor firing range.

What NIOSH Did

- We evaluated noise and lead exposures in April 2011.
- We took personal measurements for noise and lead.
- We took surface wipe samples and hand wipe samples for lead.
- We measured sound levels at different frequencies during live fire training.

What NIOSH Found

- Employee exposures to noise were above the NIOSH recommended exposure limit.
- Peak noise levels were above 160 decibels during gunfire.
- Employee exposure to lead did not exceed occupational exposure limits.
- We found lead on surfaces.
- Students appeared to have good hand washing practices.

What Managers Can Do

- Establish a hearing conservation program that includes annual audiograms for instructors.
- Require instructors and students to wear dual hearing protection during weapon fire, and provide training to ensure proper use. Dual hearing protection includes ear plugs and earmuffs.
- Consider supplying non-lead bullets and primers for classes.
- Require students and instructors to wash hands before eating, drinking, or using tobacco products.
- Notify employees and students that picnic tables have lead on them. Tell employees about the potential for getting lead from the table into their food or from their hands into their mouth. Managers should share this information with the firing range owner.

What Employees Can Do

- Wear dual hearing protection during weapon fire. Dual hearing protection includes ear plugs and earmuffs.
- Continue to use good hygiene practices. Wash your hands before eating, drinking, or using tobacco products.

Summary

Personal noise measurements taken during a basic firearms course at an outdoor firing range exceeded the NIOSH REL. Personal lead air measurements did not exceed applicable OELs, but lead was found in air samples and on a picnic table where employees ate lunch. Employees should wear double hearing protection and participate in a hearing conservation program.

On February 25, 2011, NIOSH received a technical assistance request from a federal government agency to assess exposures to noise and lead of firing range instructors at an outdoor firing range in California. On April 11–12, 2011, NIOSH investigators evaluated employee exposures to noise and lead during a 3-day basic firearms course.

Eight students and five instructors contributed 14 personal noise dosimetry measurements over 2 days. During live fire training, we measured sound levels and octave band noise frequency levels with a type 1 SLM. We took 16 PBZ air samples and six surface wipe samples for lead. We also used a colorimetric wipe test to test for lead on hands.

Noise monitoring results indicated that all participants' TWA noise exposures exceeded the NIOSH REL, some exceeded the OSHA AL, but none exceeded the OSHA PEL. However, noise dosimeter microphones and electronic circuitry do not adequately capture peak noise levels above the maximum range of the instrument, therefore, personal TWA noise measurements from gunfire noise using dosimeters should be interpreted cautiously. These measurements can underrepresent noise exposure and hearing loss risk from gunfire noise. Sound level meter measurements revealed that peak noise levels during gunfire were greater than 160 dB.

None of the lead PBZ air sampling results exceeded applicable OELs. Results varied from Day 1 to Day 2, which was likely due to the meteorological conditions. Under different meteorological conditions and employee proximity to the gun smoke source, exposures may be higher. Lead was found on the outdoor picnic table surface where we observed employees eating lunch. Employees appeared to have good hand hygiene as no lead was found on the hand wipes after washing.

Because of the high noise levels in firing ranges, double hearing protection is necessary. The noise levels generated by the firearms warrant a hearing conservation program, which should meet the requirements of the OSHA hearing conservation standard [29 CFR 1910.95]. Firing range instructors should have yearly audiometric evaluations to measure hearing levels and identify hearing loss. Reviewers of audiograms should be aware of potentiating and synergistic effects of ototoxins such as lead and solvents. To reduce lead exposures, use of non-lead bullets and non-lead primers should be considered as it becomes economically feasible. Good personal hygiene should continue to be encouraged to reduce the potential for lead ingestion.

Keywords: NAICS 922190 (Other Justice, Public Order, and Safety Activities), firearms, lead, noise, impulse noise, impulsive noise, hearing loss, shotguns, rifles, outdoor firing range, ototoxins, ototoxicity

INTRODUCTION

On February 25, 2011, NIOSH received a technical assistance request from a federal government agency to assess exposures to noise and lead among firing range instructors at an outdoor firing range in California. No employees had reported hearing loss or health concerns to management. On April 11–12, 2011, NIOSH investigators evaluated employee exposures to noise and lead during a 3-day basic firearms training course.

Firing range instructors teach 1- to 3-day basic and refresher firearm courses to other federal government employees who carry a firearm for their job. They instruct courses approximately five times a year at a rented public outdoor firing range that is closed to the public on the days the course is taught. The basic firearms course we evaluated included classroom and field practice components, with about 6 hours per day of field practice. Students completed qualifying exams on the last day of the course. The class had three to five instructors and eight students. Three instructors were always present on the firing range with the eight students. Most of the class was taught at a straight lane outdoor range where students fired at paper targets, with earth backing behind the targets. Students spread out approximately 4 feet apart in a line about 15 yards away from the targets. During live fire exercises, instructors stood about 2–3 feet behind students. Students used shotguns (12 gauge) and two types of rifles (.30-06 or .45-70) (Figure 1). Students did not use revolvers (.44 caliber) in this course, but in some other courses revolvers are also used. During the qualifying exams, students used parts of the skeet range and clay courses. The instructors selected ammunition for the course. Shotguns used rifled lead slugs. Rifles used bullets with partial or full copper metal jacket over lead. All the primers contained lead. The number of rounds fired in a typical training day varied depending on the class size and experience. Towards the end of the course, the instructors taught students how to clean the firearms.

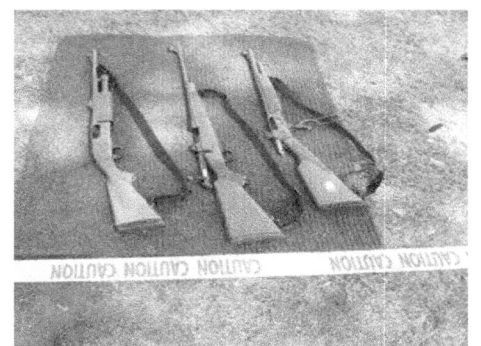

Figure 1. Firearms used for training (from left to right: 12-gauge shotgun, .30-06 rifle, and .45-70 rifle).

The instructors brought all equipment, ammunition, PPE, and teaching materials to the firing range. They did not store any of their property at the range. All instructors and students wore safety glasses and earmuffs. During our evaluation, students wore 3M (St. Paul, Minnesota) Peltor® Tactical™ 6-S with an NRR of 19 dB, and instructors wore Peltor® PowerCom Plus™ with an NRR of 25 dB during live fire. The agency had no blood lead monitoring program and no hearing conservation program although a draft hearing conservation program written by the agency safety specialist had been submitted to management. We obtained MSDSs for the chemicals used for cleaning the firearms.

ASSESSMENT

We held an opening meeting on April 11, 2011, with employer and employee representatives. On April 11 and 12, 2011, we interviewed several instructors; observed classroom and field activities; measured outdoor temperature, wind direction, and velocity; and sampled for noise and lead.

Eight students and five instructors contributed 14 personal noise dosimetry measurements over 2 days. Students and instructors wore integrating noise dosimeters on Day 1 of sampling. However, only instructors wore dosimeters on Day 2 of sampling. We measured area noise levels and performed octave band frequency spectrum analysis (measurement of noise levels in different frequencies) with two SLM and real-time frequency analyzers. The SLMs were mounted on tripods at a height of approximately 5 feet to represent the ear position of a standing shooter. We placed the tripods with SLMs on each end of the firing line approximately 4 to 6 feet from the student (Figure 2). Because of safety concerns and risk of interfering with students and instructors, we were not able to place SLMs closer during live fire training sessions. However, during some of the qualifying exams, we handheld the SLMs approximately 1 to 2 feet from the instructor's ear.

We took 16 personal breathing zone air samples and six surface wipe samples for lead. Surfaces tested included areas that people frequently touched, such as the trigger and forend of the firearm, doorknobs, and restroom water faucet handles. We also used a colorimetric wipe test to test for lead on hands.

More information on OELs and health effects for noise and lead can be found in Appendix A. More information on sampling methodology for noise and lead can be found in Appendix B.

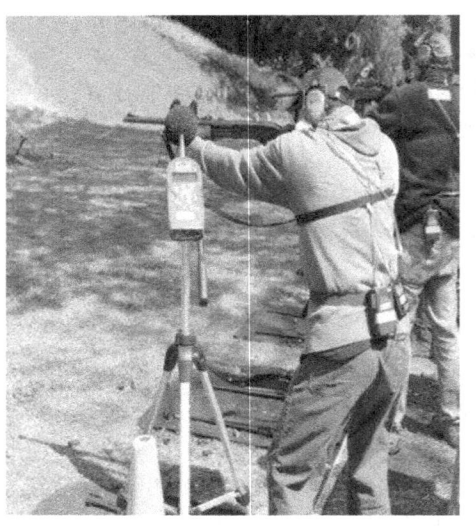

Figure 2. Sound level meter at firing line during firearm training exercises.

RESULTS AND DISCUSSION

Noise

Results from the personal dosimetry measurements are provided in Table 1. Results indicated that all participants' TWA noise exposures exceeded the NIOSH REL, some exceeded the OSHA AL, but none exceeded the OSHA PEL. Noise dosimeter microphones and electronic circuitry do not adequately capture peak noise levels above the maximum range of the instrument and "clip" noise levels at approximately 145 dB. Previous research on the use of dosimeters for gunfire measurements concluded that these electroacoustic limitations produce errors in calculating TWA noise levels from impulsive noise environments [Kardous et al. 2003; Kardous and Willson 2004]. Therefore, personal TWA noise measurements from gunfire noise collected with dosimeters should be interpreted cautiously and considered to underrepresent noise exposure and hearing loss risk from gunfire noise.

Table 1. Personal noise dosimetry results*

Job title	Duration	OSHA AL			OSHA PEL			NIOSH REL		
	(h:mm)	TWA†	TWA 8-hr‡	Dose§	TWA†	TWA 8-hr‡	Dose§	TWA†	TWA 8-hr‡	Dose§
		(dBA)	(dBA)	(%)	(dBA)	(dBA)	(%)	(dBA)	(dBA)	(%)
Student	5:00	*89*	*85*	*50*	89	85	50	*100*	*97*	*1598*
Student	4:54	87	84	44	87	84	44	*99*	*96*	*1269*
Student	4:59	88	84	44	87	84	44	*98*	*96*	*1269*
Student	5:04	86	82	33	86	82	33	*97*	*95*	*1007*
Student	4:52	86	83	38	86	82	33	*98*	*95*	*1007*
Student	4:57	84	80	25	84	80	25	*95*	*93*	*634*
Instructor	4:59	*89*	*85*	*50*	88	84	44	*98*	*96*	*1269*
Instructor	4:53	*89*	*86*	*57*	88	85	50	*96*	*94*	*799*
Instructor	4:55	82	78	19	82	78	19	*93*	*91*	*400*
Instructor	5:37	*88*	*85*	*50*	87	85	50	*97*	*96*	*1269*
Instructor	4:59	86	83	38	86	83	38	*97*	*95*	*1007*
Instructor	5:42	84	82	33	84	81	29	*95*	*94*	*799*
Instructor	6:30	83	82	33	82	80	25	*95*	*94*	*799*
Instructor	6:34	78	75	13	78	74	11	*90*	*88*	*200*
Exposure Limits		85	50		90	100		85	100	

* Exposures at or exceeding exposure limits are highlighted in bold and italicized font.
† TWA noise exposures for the duration of the noise monitoring period
‡ Projected 8-hour TWA assuming that noise exposures beyond the measured duration were below 80 dBA
§ Dose is based on TWA 8-hour noise exposure.

RESULTS AND DISCUSSION
(CONTINUED)

One-third octave band noise frequency measurements collected when students were shooting .45-70 rifles are shown in Figure 3. These measurements showed that the highest sound pressure levels (125 dB) occurred at 500 Hz, and were greater than 110 dB across all the one-third octave bands from 125 Hz to 20,000 Hz. Measurements taken during shooting of the 12-gauge shotgun and the .30-06 rifle had similar results. Octave band measurements provide information about the frequency distribution of noise. Because the energy from noise is usually widely distributed over many frequencies, the frequency range is broken into a smaller range of frequencies (called bandwidths), the most common being the octave band (defined as a frequency band where the upper band frequency is twice the lower band-edge frequency).

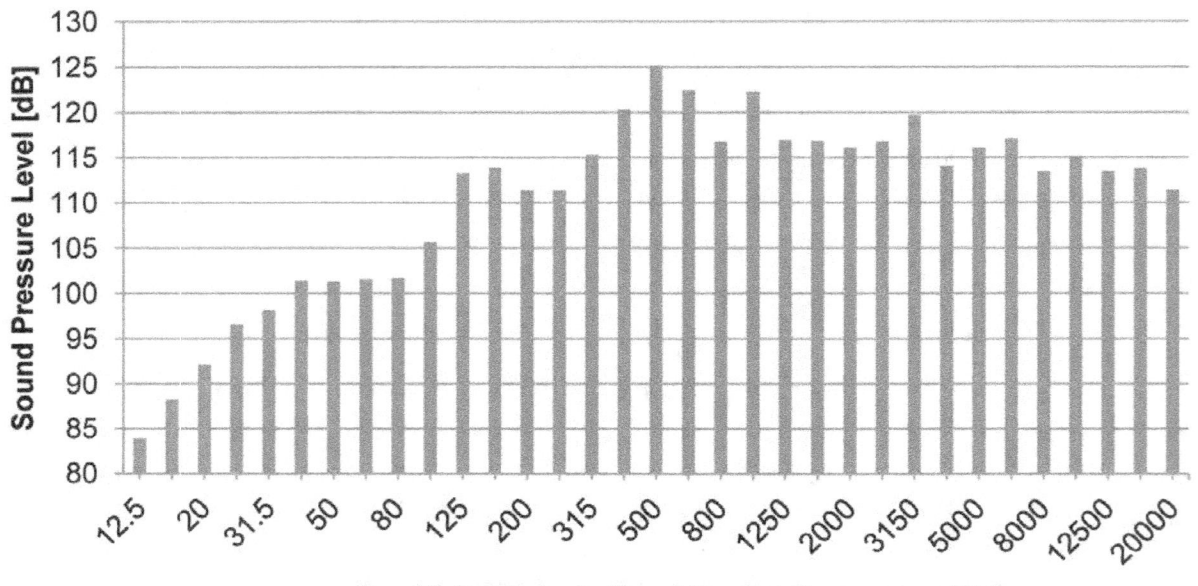

Figure 3. One-third octave band noise frequency levels of four rifles (.45-70) being fired over a 90-second period during a basic firearms training course.

Octave band analysis allows for determination of the dominant noise frequencies and can be useful for identifying potential engineering controls. For example, if low frequency noise is dominant (i.e., the highest octave-band sound levels occur in frequencies of 500 Hz or less), noise is likely generated by vibration, and noise controls that reduce or isolate the vibration from tools or equipment might decrease noise levels. If high frequency noise is dominant (i.e., the highest octave band sound levels occur in frequencies of 2,000 Hz or greater), noise enclosures, barriers, or sound absorption systems are typically the most effective approach [Driscoll and Royster 2003]. One of the

RESULTS AND DISCUSSION
(CONTINUED)

primary sources of noise generated during gunfire is the muzzle blast during firing, which generates high noise across the mid to high frequency range. The only potentially effective noise control method to reduce students' or instructors' noise exposure from gunfire is through the use of noise suppressors that can be attached to the end of the gun barrel. However, some states do not permit civilians to use suppressors on firearms.

Peak sound levels ranged from 154.6 dB to 163.1 dB during shooting exercises. Peak levels for the 12-gauge shotgun and .30-06 rifles were slightly higher than for the .45-70 rifle (Table 2). During training exercises, students typically fire a series of shots in succession followed by several minutes without shooting for instruction. An example of peak sound levels during 1 minute of shooting a .30-06 rifle is shown in Figure 4. Eight peaks greater than 160 dB and several others greater than 150 dB can be seen during this time period.

Table 2. Peak sound level range for firearms

Firearm	Peak Sound Level Range (dB)	Ammunition Weight (Grains)
12-Gauge Shotgun	154.6 – 162.7	438
.45-70 Rifle	155.2 – 159.9	350
.30-06 Rifle	158.7 – 163.1	173

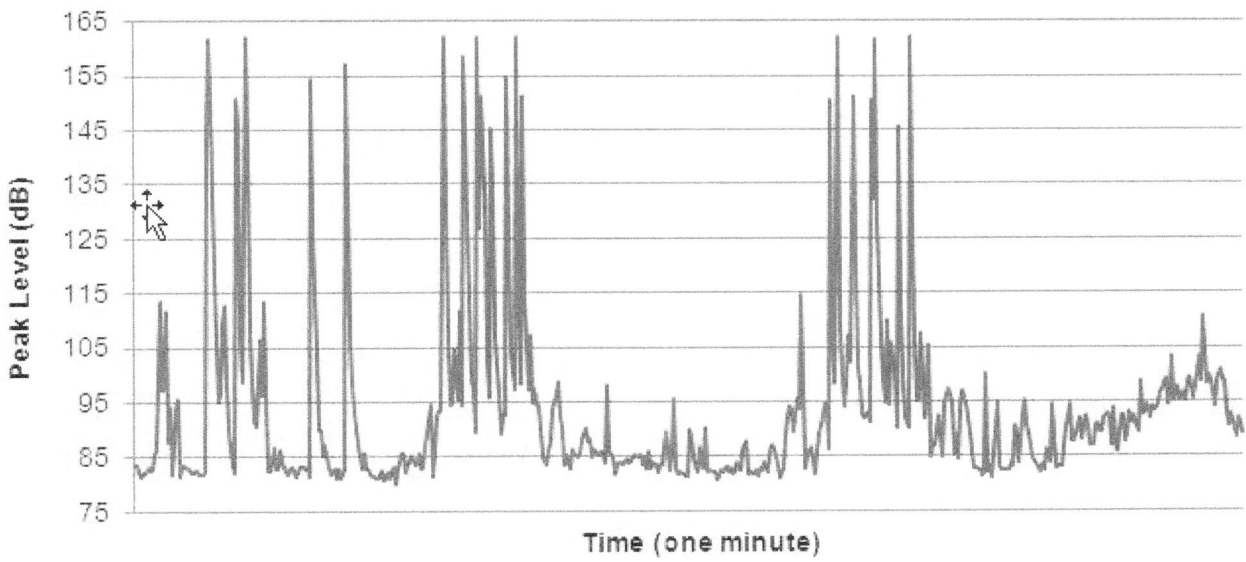

Figure 4. Peak sound levels during one minute of shooting .30-06 rifles in a training exercise.

Research has shown that repeated exposure to impulse noise can result in permanent NIHL [Patterson and Hamernik 1992; Pekkarinen et al. 1993; Chan et al. 2001]. Noise produced by impulsive noise, such as gunfire, has sufficient intensity to permanently damage unprotected ears in a very short period of time; damage can occur in minutes rather than the days or years typical of industrial noise exposure. The OSHA PEL and NIOSH REL state that exposure to impulse noise should not exceed 140 dB. However, peak impulse is not the sole factor in hearing damage. Other factors such as duration of the impulse and frequency of exposure also have an effect on hearing loss.

Because of the high noise levels in firing ranges, double hearing protection is necessary to protect hearing. Research has reported that double hearing protection can provide the additional noise reduction needed in high noise level environments [Berger 1983]. However, proper insertion of hearing protection is critically important to ensure proper noise attenuation. NIOSH has previously identified poor insertion of formable hearing protection into the ear canals [NIOSH 2005].

To estimate hearing protector attenuation NIOSH recommends using subject fit data based on the American National Standards Institute's standard S12.6-1997 [ANSI 1997]. However, if no subject fit data are available, NIOSH recommends adjusting the hearing protectors' ratings by subtracting 25% from the manufacturer's labeled NRR for earmuffs and subtracting 50% from the manufacturer's labeled NRR for formable earplugs. An additional 5 to 10 dB of attenuation can be added for use of dual hearing protection [NIOSH 1998]. Figure 5 shows the range of estimated noise attenuation that could be achieved for properly fitted and worn ear plugs and earmuffs, using NIOSH noise attenuation calculations for unweighted or dBC noise exposure levels. For dBA noise exposure levels, an additional 7 dB should be subtracted from the derated NRR.

On the basis of hearing protection worn by instructors and students during the training class (instructors: Peltor® PowerCon Plus™ with an NRR of 25 dB; students: Peltor® Tactical™ 6-S with an NRR of 19 dB), the estimated hearing protector attenuation using the NIOSH hearing protector derating formula is 19 dB for instructors and 14 dB for students. If instructors and students wore earmuffs with an NRR of 33 dB along with properly inserted ear plugs, their estimated attenuation for dual

RESULTS AND DISCUSSION
(CONTINUED)

protection using the NIOSH hearing protector derating formula would increase to 30–35 dB. In tests of hearing protection using an acoustic mannequin, NIOSH found that in some instances double hearing protection actually provided more peak noise attenuation than the NIOSH hearing protector derating formula calculates [NIOSH 2003, 2005].

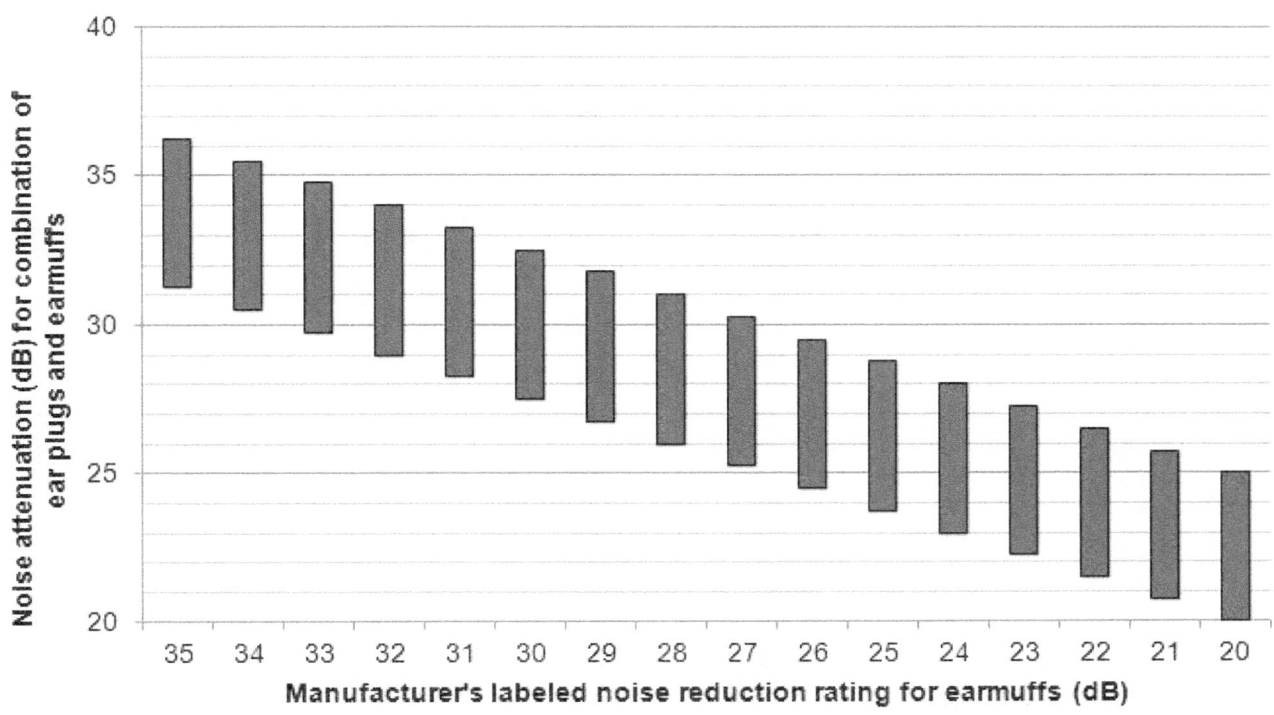

Figure 5. Range of estimated noise attenuation (dB) for combination of properly fitted and worn insert type ear plugs and earmuffs, based on NIOSH noise attenuation calculations for unweighted or dBC noise levels.

In 2002, NIOSH proposed a simplified formula to reduce the risk of exposure to impulse noise in terms of the number of gunshot impulses to which a person can be exposed per day [NIOSH 2002]:

$$N = 10^{((140 - PI)/10)}$$

where N is the number of gunshot exposures permitted, and PI is the peak impulse level in dB under hearing protection. PI is determined by subtracting the noise attenuation for hearing protection from the peak noise exposure level for a gunfire impulse.

Figure 6 shows the number of gunshot exposures permitted on the basis of peak noise levels under hearing protection. For example, if the peak noise level under hearing protection is 120 dB, applying this formula yields N=100 gunshots. The NIOSH proposed formula is a conservative estimate and does not take into account the duration of the impulse, its spectral content, or its energy.

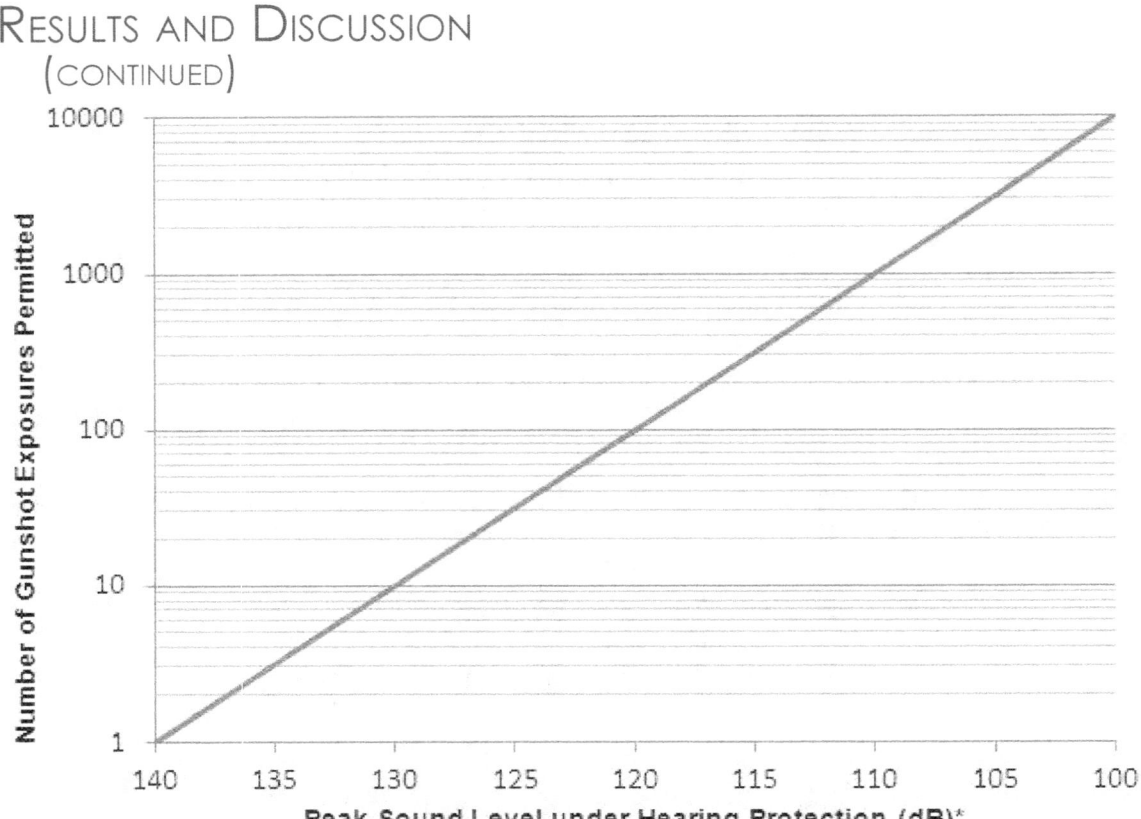

*Peak sound level under hearing protection is calculated by subtracting the estimated noise attenuation for hearing protection from the peak noise exposure level for a gunfire impulse.

Figure 6. Number of gunshot exposures permitted using NIOSH recommendations [NIOSH 2002], based on peak sound levels (dB) under hearing protection.

Lead

We collected 16 PBZ area air samples on students and instructors for lead. None of our results exceeded applicable OELs. These results are listed in Table 3. Results from Day 1 were very low with only one quantifiable PBZ air sample. Results from Day 2 were higher than Day 1, with the highest lead exposure found on an instructor at 15 µg/m³. The concentration differences between Day 1 and Day 2 were most likely due to the meteorological conditions. On Day 1, the wind moved gun smoke down the course and away from the employees. On Day 2, the wind was mild and moved gun smoke up the course towards the employees. On Day 2, it is possible that students' exposures would have been even higher than the instructors' because of their closer proximity to the smoke sources. Past studies looking at lead exposure to outdoor firearm instructors found that despite "natural ventilation" at outdoor firing ranges, PBZ levels exceeded OSHA, NIOSH, and ACGIH

RESULTS AND DISCUSSION
(CONTINUED)

OELs of 50 µg/m³ as an 8-hour TWA [Goldberg et al. 1991; Tripathi et al. 1991; Mancuso et al. 2008]. Studies have also shown that jacketed or non-lead bullets can reduce lead concentrations [NIOSH 1986; Tripathi et al. 1991; NIOSH 1995] in air and on surfaces. Although we did not find air lead levels that exceeded the OELs, it is possible that airborne lead levels could be higher during certain meteorological conditions, and care should be taken to minimize lead exposures.

Table 3. PBZ air sampling results for lead*

Day	Type	Sampling Time (min)	Sample Volume (m³)	8-hr TWA* Concentration (µg/m³)
1	Student	307	0.61	1.02
1	Student	302	0.59	[0.82]
1	Student	300	0.59	[0.75]
1	Student	306	0.60	[0.70]
1	Student	303	0.60	[0.57]
1	Student	307	0.61	[0.51]
1	Student	267	0.53	[0.44]
1	Student	304	0.60	[0.49]
1	Instructor	305	0.60	ND
1	Instructor	300	0.59	ND
2	Instructor	370	0.72	15
2	Instructor	364	0.70	4.3
2	Instructor	313	0.61	1.5
2	Instructor	359	0.70	1.2
2	Instructor	315	0.62	[0.66]
2	Instructor	297	0.58	ND
MDC†				0.32
MQC†				1.3
NIOSH REL (8-hr TWA)				50
OSHA PEL (8-hr TWA)				50
ACGIH TLV (8-hr TWA)				50

Values in brackets indicate levels between the MDC and MQC.

*Concentrations were calculated to reflect an 8-hour TWA by assuming no lead exposure beyond the measured duration.

†Based on an air volume of 0.62 m³.

RESULTS AND DISCUSSION
(CONTINUED)

The highest levels of surface contamination for lead were found on the firearms, which was expected (Table 4). Lead levels were much lower on surfaces where frequent contact occurs, such as door and sink handles. Lead was found on the outdoor picnic table surface where we observed employees eating lunch, so care should be taken to prevent lead from transferring from the table surface to food or hands to mouth.

Table 4. Lead surface wipe sampling results

Location	Concentration (µg/100 cm²)
Rifle forend*	1.0
Shotgun stock*	0.68
Rifle stock*	0.10
Picnic table	0.08
Men's restroom sink handles*	0.03
Door handle into classroom*	0.02

* Approximated 100 cm² surface area

All students showed a positive result for lead on their hands immediately after returning from the range after live firearms practice. After hand washing, no positive result was observed on the hand wipes (Figure 7). We also asked one instructor to use the wipes after returning from the range and washing hands. The instructor's hand wipe results showed a negative result. Aside from an occasional demonstration, the instructors did not usually handle firearms. These results indicate that students had good hand hygiene.

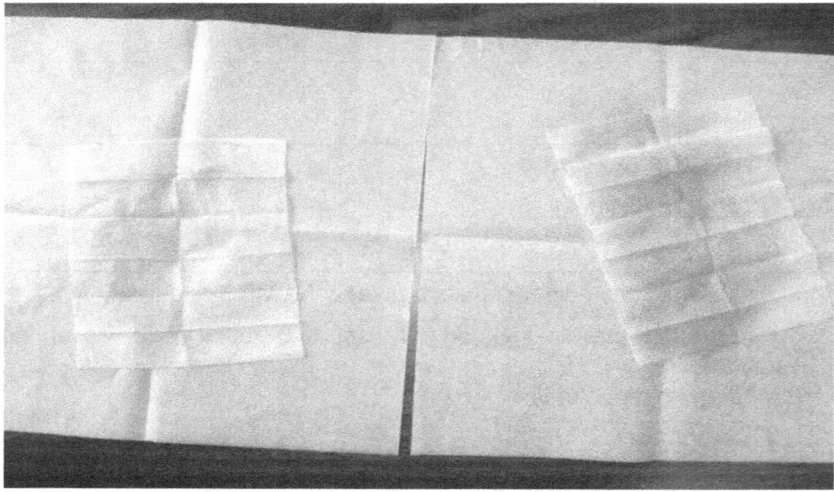

Figure 7. The left wipe, taken from a student who had just returned from the shooting range and had not yet washed hands, is positive for lead. The right wipe, taken after the student had washed hands, is negative for lead.

Health Hazard Evaluation Report 2011-0069-3140

Ototoxins

Ototoxins are chemicals that can cause hearing damage when absorbed into the body. Studies have shown that exposure to some chemicals, such as lead and some solvents, can cause hearing loss [Sliwinska-Kowalska et al. 2004; Hwang et al. 2009]. The mechanism of loss is not well understood, but it is hypothesized that ototoxins entering the blood stream damage inner ear structures, causing nerve damage and/or oxidative stress [Henderson et al 2006; Johnson and Morata 2010]. Some chemicals may not cause hearing loss alone, but can exacerbate hearing loss caused by noise (potentiation). Some chemicals may cause a synergistic effect, where the combined effect of the two exposures is greater than either alone. It is difficult to distinguish whether hearing loss is caused by ototoxicants or excessive noise, as both losses appear similar on pure tone audiograms and have many other similar characteristics (e.g., bilateral loss, loss starting in the high frequencies).

Solvents are used to clean firearms after use. Although none of the ingredients listed on the MSDS that were given to us had been observed as ototoxicants, users should be aware that moderate exposures (below or around the OEL) to solvents such as toluene [Morata et al. 1993; Chang et al. 2006], xylene, and mixtures of solvents [Sliwinska-Kowalska et al. 2004; Fuente et al. 2009] have been shown to be associated with hearing loss [Sliwinska-Kowalska et al. 2007].

The ACGIH states that, "In settings where there may be exposures to noise and to carbon monoxide, lead, manganese styrene, toluene, or xylene, periodic audiograms are advised and should be carefully reviewed" [ACGIH 2011]. The U.S. Army recommends annual audiometric monitoring when workers are exposed to air concentrations that are at or exceed 50% of the most stringent OEL criteria for a variety of ototoxicants including solvents and lead [U.S. Army 2009]. The highest lead PBZ air concentration (15 mg/m^3) did not exceed 50% of the NIOSH REL, but because meteorological factors may cause variations in worker exposure, it is possible that exposure on a different day could be higher. We were also told that some instructors shot recreationally, which would contribute to their overall lead and noise exposures. Reviewers of employees' audiometric tests should be aware of possible additive, potentiating, or synergistic effects between noise exposure, solvents, and lead when evaluating audiograms.

CONCLUSIONS

Personal noise measurements taken during a basic firearms course exceeded the NIOSH REL, some exceeded the OSHA AL, but none exceeded the OSHA PEL. Peak sound levels exceeded 160 dB. Because of the high noise levels in shooting ranges, the use of double hearing protection is necessary. The noise levels generated by the firearms warrant a hearing conservation program, and firing range instructors should have yearly audiometric evaluations. Personal lead air measurements did not exceed applicable OELs, but lead was observed in the air and on some surfaces. Meteorological conditions and employee proximity to the gun smoke may greatly affect exposures. Reviewers of audiograms should be aware of potentiating and synergistic effects of ototoxins. To reduce lead exposures, use of non-lead bullets and non-lead primers as they become economically feasible should be considered. Good personal hygiene should be encouraged to reduce lead ingestion potential.

RECOMMENDATIONS

On the basis of our findings, we recommend the actions listed below to create a more healthful workplace. Our recommendations are based on the hierarchy of controls approach (refer to Appendix A: Occupational Exposure Limits and Health Effects). This approach groups actions by their likely effectiveness in reducing or removing hazards. In most cases, the preferred approach is to eliminate hazardous materials or processes and install engineering controls to reduce exposure or shield employees. Until such controls are in place, or if they are not effective or feasible, administrative measures and/or personal protective equipment may be needed. PPE is the least effective means for controlling employee exposures. Proper use of PPE requires a comprehensive program, and calls for a high level of employee involvement and commitment to be effective.

1. The noise levels generated by the firearms warrant a hearing conservation program. At a minimum, the program should meet the requirements of the OSHA hearing conservation standard [29 CFR 1910.95]. Another source for designing an effective hearing loss prevention program is the NIOSH occupational noise criteria document [NIOSH 1998].

2. Firing range instructors should have yearly audiometric evaluations to measure hearing levels and identify hearing loss. Reviewers of audiograms should be aware of potentiating and synergistic effects of ototoxins, such as lead and solvents, on hearing loss.

RECOMMENDATIONS

(CONTINUED)

3. Instructors and students should wear dual hearing protection (ear plugs and earmuffs) during weapons fire. For maximum protection, select earmuffs and ear plugs that provide a high level of noise attenuation. Because of the critical importance of proper use and fit, train students and instructors how to properly wear hearing protection. Encourage the use of dual hearing protection during recreational shooting.

4. Consider using non-lead bullets and non-lead primers as they become economically feasible.

5. Employees should follow safe work practices identified by the firing range and employer. They should continue good personal hygiene practices including hand washing before eating, drinking, smoking, and leaving the range.

6. Assume that picnic tables are contaminated with lead, and take precautions to prevent transfer of lead from surface to food or hands to mouth (e.g , cover the table with a disposable tablecloth before eating). This information should be shared with the range owner.

REFERENCES

ACGIH [2011]. 2011 TLVs® and BEIs®: threshold limit values for chemical substances and physical agents and biological exposure indices. Cincinnati, OH: American Conference of Governmental Industrial Hygienists.

ANSI [1997]. American national standard: methods for measuring the real-ear attenuation of hearing protectors. New York: American National Standards Institute, Inc. ANSI S12.6-1997.

Berger EH [1983]. Laboratory attenuation of earmuffs and earplugs both singly and in combination. Am Ind Hyg Assoc J 44(5):321–329.

CFR. Code of Federal Regulations. Washington, DC: U.S. Government Printing Office, Office of the Federal Register.

Chan PC, Ho KH, Kan KK, Stuhmiller JH, Mayorga MA [2001]. Evaluation of impulse noise criteria using human volunteer data. J Acoust Soc Amer 110(4):1967–1975.

Chang SJ, Chen CJ, Lien CH, Sung FC [2006]. Hearing loss in workers exposed to toluene and noise. Environ Health Perspect 114(8):1283–1286.

Driscoll DP, Royster LH [2003]. Noise control engineering. In: Berger EH, Royster LH, Royster JD, Driscoll DP, Layne M. eds, The noise manual, 5th ed. Akron, OH: American Industrial Hygiene Association, pp. 279–378; [Reference: Table 9.5, pp. 298–300].

Fuente A, Slade MD, Taylor T, Morata TC, Keith RW, Sparer J, Rabinowitz PM [2009]. Peripheral and central auditory dysfunction induced by occupational exposure to organic solvents. J Occup Environ Med 51(10):1202–1211.

Goldberg RL, Hicks AM, O'Leary LM, London S [1991]. Lead exposures at uncovered outdoor firing ranges. J Occup Med 33(6):718–719.

Henderson D, Bielefeld EC, Harris KC, Hu BH [2006]. The role of oxidative stress in noise-induced hearing loss. Ear Hear 27(1):1–19.

Hwang YH, Chiang HY, Yen-Jean MC, Wang JD [2009]. The association between low levels of lead in blood and occupational noise-induced hearing loss in steel workers. Sci Total Environ 408(1):43–49.

References
(CONTINUED)

Johnson A, Morata TC [2010]. Occupational exposure to chemicals and hearing impairment. In: The Nordic expert group for criteria documentation of health risks from chemicals. Kjell Torén, ed. Gothenburg, Sweden. pp. 14–19.

Kardous CA, Willson RD, Hayden CS, Szlapa P, Murphy WJ, Reeves ER [2003]. Noise exposure assessment and abatement strategies at an indoor firing range. App Occ Environ Hyg 18(8):629–636.

Kardous CA, Willson RD [2004]. Limitations of using dosimeters in impulse noise environments. J Occup Environ Hyg 1(7):456–462.

Mancuso JD, McCoy J, Pelka B, Kahn PJ, Gaydos JC [2008]. The challenge of controlling lead and silica exposures from firing ranges in a special operations force. Military Med 173(2):182–186.

Morata TC, Dunn DE, Kretschmer LW, Lemasters GK, Keith RW [1993]. Effects of occupational exposure to organic solvents and noise on hearing. Scand J Work Environ Health 19(4):245–254.

NIOSH [1986]. Hazard evaluation and technical assistance report: Federal reserve bank, Cincinnati, OH. By Lee S. Cincinnati, OH: U.S. Department of Health and Human Services, Centers for Disease Control and Prevention, National Institute for Occupational Safety and Health, HETA Report No. 86-0269-1812.

NIOSH [1995]. Hazard evaluation and technical assistance report: Colorado state patrol training academy, Golden, Colorado. By Lee S and Boudreau Y. Cincinnati, OH: U.S. Department of Health and Human Services, Centers for Disease Control and Prevention, National Institute for Occupational Safety and Health, HETA Report No. 95-0290-9221.

NIOSH [1998]. Criteria for a recommended standard: occupational noise exposure (revised criteria 1998). Cincinnati, OH: U.S. Department of Health and Human Services, Centers for Disease Control and Prevention, National Institute for Occupational Safety and Health, DHHS (NIOSH) Publication No. 98-126.

NIOSH [2002]. Comments of the National Institute for Occupational Safety and Health on the Occupational Safety and Health Administration ANPR Hearing Conservation Program for Construction Workers 29 CFR Part 1926 Docket No. H–011G. Cincinnati, OH: U.S. Department of Health and Human Services, Centers for Disease Control and Prevention, National Institute for Occupational Safety and Health.

NIOSH [2003]. Hazard evaluation and technical assistance report: Fort Collins Police Services, Fort Collins, CO. By Tubbs R, Murphy W. Cincinnati, OH: U.S. Department of Health and Human Services, Centers for Disease Control and Prevention, National Institute for Occupational Safety and Health, NIOSH HETA Report No. 2002-0131-2898.

NIOSH [2005]. Hazard evaluation and technical assistance report: Immigration and naturalization service, National Firearms Unit, Altoona, PA. By Harney J, King B, Tubbs R, Crouch K, Hayden C, Kardous C, Khan A, Mickelsen L, Willson R. Cincinnati, OH: U.S. Department of Health and Human Services, Centers for Disease Control and Prevention, National Institute for Occupational Safety and Health, HETA Report No. 2000-0191-2960.

Patterson J, Hamernik R [1992]. An experimental basis for the estimation of auditory system following exposures to impulse noise. In: Noise-induced hearing loss. Dancer A, Henderson D, Salvi R, Hamernik R, eds. Philadelphia, PA: BC Decker, pp. 336–348.

Pekkarinen J, Iki M, Starck J, Pyykko I [1993]. Hearing loss risk from exposure to shooting impulses in workers exposed to occupational noise. Br J Aud 27(3):175–182.

Sliwinska-Kowalska M, Zamyslowska-Szmytke E, Szymczak W, Kotylo P, Fiszer M, Wesolowski W, Pawlaczyk-Luszczynska M, Bak M, Gajda-Szadkowska A [2004]. Effects of coexposure to noise and mixture of organic solvents on hearing in dockyard workers. J Occup Environ Med 46(1):30–38.

Sliwinska-Kowalska M, Prasher D, Rodrigues CA, Zamyslowska-Szmytke E, Campo P, Henderson D, Lund SP, Johnson AC, Schäper M, Odkvist L, Starck J, Toppila E, Schneider E, Möller C, Fuente A, Gopal KV [2007]. Ototoxicity of organic solvents - from scientific evidence to health policy. Int J Occup Med Environ Hlth 20(2):215–22.

Tripathi RK, Sheretz PC, Llewellyn GS, Armstrong CW [1991]. Lead exposure in outdoor firearm instructors. Am J Pub Hlth 81(6):753–755.

U.S. Army [2009] Just the facts...Occupational ototoxins (ear poisons) and hearing loss. Hearing Conservation and Industrial Hygiene and Medical Safety Management [http://www.nmcphc.med.navy.mil/downloads/occmed/toolbox/occupationalototoxinfactsheet-chppm.pdf]. Date accessed: July 2011.

In evaluating the hazards posed by workplace exposures, NIOSH investigators use both mandatory (legally enforceable) and recommended OELs for chemical, physical, and biological agents as a guide for making recommendations. OELs have been developed by federal agencies and safety and health organizations to prevent the occurrence of adverse health effects from workplace exposures. Generally, OELs suggest levels of exposure that most employees may be exposed to for up to 10 hours per day, 40 hours per week, for a working lifetime, without experiencing adverse health effects. However, not all employees will be protected from adverse health effects even if their exposures are maintained below these levels. A small percentage may experience adverse health effects because of individual susceptibility, a preexisting medical condition, and/or a hypersensitivity (allergy). In addition, some hazardous substances may act in combination with other workplace exposures, the general environment, or with medications or personal habits of the employee to produce adverse health effects even if the occupational exposures are controlled at the level set by the exposure limit. Also, some substances can be absorbed by direct contact with the skin and mucous membranes in addition to being inhaled, which contributes to the individual's overall exposure.

Most OELs are expressed as a TWA exposure. A TWA refers to the average exposure during a normal 8- to 10-hour workday. In the United States, OELs have been established by federal agencies, professional organizations, state and local governments, and other entities. Some OELs are legally enforceable limits, while others are recommendations. The U.S. Department of Labor OSHA PELs (29 CFR 1910 [general industry]; 29 CFR 1926 [construction industry]; and 29 CFR 1917 [maritime industry]) are legal limits enforceable in workplaces covered under the Occupational Safety and Health Act of 1970. NIOSH RELs are recommendations based on a critical review of the scientific and technical information available on a given hazard and the adequacy of methods to identify and control the hazard. NIOSH RELs can be found in the NIOSH Pocket Guide to Chemical Hazards [NIOSH 2010]. NIOSH also recommends different types of risk management practices (e.g., engineering controls, safe work practices, employee education/training, personal protective equipment, and exposure and medical monitoring) to minimize the risk of exposure and adverse health effects from these hazards. Other OELs that are commonly used and cited in the United States include the TLVs recommended by ACGIH, a professional organization, and the WEELs recommended by the AIHA, another professional organization. The TLVs and WEELs are developed by committee members of these associations from a review of the published, peer-reviewed literature. They are not consensus standards. ACGIH TLVs are considered voluntary exposure guidelines for use by industrial hygienists and others trained in this discipline "to assist in the control of health hazards" [ACGIH 2011]. WEELs have been established for some chemicals "when no other legal or authoritative limits exist" [AIHA 2011].

Outside the United States, OELs have been established by various agencies and organizations and include both legal and recommended limits. The Institut für Arbeitsschutz der Deutschen Gesetzlichen Unfallversicherung (IFA, Institute for Occupational Safety and Health of the German Social Accident Insurance) maintains a database of international OELs from European Union member states, Canada (Québec), Japan, Switzerland, and the United States. The database, available at http://www.dguv.de/ifa/en/gestis/limit_values/index.jsp, contains international limits for over 1,500 hazardous substances and is updated periodically.

NIOSH investigators encourage the use of the traditional hierarchy of controls approach to eliminate or minimize identified workplace hazards. This includes, in order of preference, the use of (1) substitution or elimination of the hazardous agent, (2) engineering controls (e.g., local exhaust ventilation, process enclosure, dilution ventilation), (3) administrative controls (e.g , limiting time of exposure, employee training, work practice changes, medical surveillance), and (4) personal protective equipment (e.g., respiratory protection, gloves, eye protection, hearing protection).

Below we provide the OELs and surface contamination limits for the compounds we measured, as well as a discussion of the potential health effects from exposure to these compounds.

Lead

Lead is ubiquitous in U.S. urban environments due to the widespread use of lead compounds in industry, gasoline, and paints during the past century. Exposure to lead occurs via inhalation of dust and fume and via ingestion through contact with lead-contaminated hands, food, cigarettes, and clothing. Absorbed lead accumulates in the body in the soft tissues and bones. Lead is stored in bones for decades, and may cause health effects long after exposure as it is slowly released in the body.

Symptoms of chronic lead poisoning include headache, joint and muscle aches, weakness, fatigue, irritability, depression, constipation, anorexia, and abdominal discomfort [Moline and Landrigan 2005]. Overexposure to lead may also result in kidney damage, anemia, high blood pressure, infertility and reduced sex drive in both sexes, and impotence. In most cases, an individual's BLL is a good indication of recent exposure to lead, with a half-life (the time interval it takes for the quantity in the body to be reduced by half its initial value) of 1-2 months [Lauwerys and Hoet 2001; Moline and Landrigan 2005; NCEH 2005]. Elevated zinc protoporphyrin levels have also been used as an indicator of chronic lead intoxication, however, other factors, such as iron deficiency, can cause an elevated zinc protoporphyrin level, so the BLL is a more specific test for evaluating occupational lead exposure.

Under the OSHA general industry lead standard (29 CFR 1910.1025), the PEL for airborne exposure to lead is 50 $\mu g/m^3$ for an 8-hour TWA. The standard requires lowering the PEL for shifts exceeding 8 hours, medical monitoring for employees exposed to airborne lead at or above the AL of 30 $\mu g/m^3$ (8-hour TWA), medical removal of employees whose average BLL is 50 $\mu g/dL$ or greater, and economic protection for medically removed workers. Medically removed workers cannot return to jobs involving lead exposure until their BLL is below 40 $\mu g/dL$. NIOSH has an REL for lead of 50 $\mu g/m^3$ averaged over an 8-hour work shift [NIOSH 2010]. ACGIH has a TLV for lead of 50 $\mu g/m^3$ (8-hour TWA), with worker BLLs to be controlled to or below 30 $\mu g/dL$, and designation of lead as an animal carcinogen [ACGIH 2011].

The NIOSH REL is consistent with the OSHA PEL, which is intended to maintain worker BLLs below 40 $\mu g/dL$. This is also intended to prevent overt symptoms of lead poisoning, but is not sufficient to protect workers from more subtle adverse health effects like hypertension, renal dysfunction, and reproductive and cognitive effects [Schwartz and Stewart 2007; Schwartz and Hu 2007; Brown-Williams et al. 2009]. Adverse effects on the adult reproductive, cardiovascular, and hematologic systems, and on the development of children of exposed workers, can occur at BLLs as low as 10 $\mu g/dL$ [Sussell 1998]. Recommendations from the March 2007 edition of Environmental Health Perspectives' Mini-Monograph on adult lead exposure and from the Association of Occupational and Environmental Clinics include advising workers and shooters that BLLs should be kept below 10 $\mu g/dL$ [CSTE 2009].

In homes with a family member occupationally exposed to lead, care must be taken to prevent "take home" of lead, that is, lead carried into the home on clothing, skin, hair, and in vehicles. High BLLs in resident children and elevated concentrations of lead in the house dust have been found in the homes of workers employed in industries associated with high lead exposure [Grandjean and Bach 1986]. Particular effort should be made to ensure that children of persons who work in areas of high lead exposure receive a BLL test. The current CDC screening guidelines for children use 10 $\mu g/dL$ as a "level of concern" in order to intervene and prevent long-term cognitive deficits [CDC 2005].

Lead-contaminated surface dust represents a potential source of lead exposure, particularly for young children. This may occur either by direct hand-to-mouth contact, or indirectly from hand-to-mouth contact with contaminated clothing, cigarettes, or food. Previous studies have found a significant correlation between resident children's BLLs and house dust lead levels [Farfel and Chisholm 1990]. In the workplace, generally there is little or no correlation between surface lead levels and employee exposures because ingestion exposures are highly dependent on personal hygiene practices and available facilities for maintaining personal hygiene. No current federal standard provides a permissible limit for lead contamination of surfaces in occupational settings.

Noise

Noise-induced hearing loss is an irreversible, sensorineural condition that progresses with exposure. Although hearing ability declines with age (presbycusis), noise exposure produces more hearing loss than that resulting from aging alone. This NIHL is caused by damage to nerve cells of the inner ear (cochlea) and, unlike some conductive hearing disorders, cannot be treated medically [Berger et al. 2003]. In most cases, NIHL develops slowly and usually occurs before it is noticed. Hearing loss is often severe enough to permanently affect a person's ability to hear and understand speech. For example, people with hearing loss may not be able to distinguish words such as "fish" from "fist." [Suter 1978].

The dBA is the preferred unit for measuring sound levels to assess employee noise exposures. The dBA noise scale is weighted to approximate the sensory response of human ears to sound frequencies near the hearing threshold. Because the dBA scale is logarithmic, increases of 3 dBA, 10 dBA, and 20 dBA represent a doubling, tenfold increase, and hundredfold increase of sound energy, respectively. Noise exposures expressed in dBA cannot be averaged by taking the arithmetic mean.

The OSHA noise standard [29 CFR 1910.95] specifies a PEL of 90 dBA as an 8-hour TWA. The OSHA PEL is calculated using a 5 dB exchange rate. This means that a person may be exposed to noise levels of 95 dBA for no more than 4 hours, 100 dBA for 2 hours, 105 dBA for 1 hour, etc. An employee's daily noise dose, on the basis of duration and intensity of noise exposure, can be calculated according to the formula:

$$Dose = 100 \times (C1/T1 + C2/T2 + ... + Cn/Tn),$$

where Cn indicates the total time of exposure at a specific noise level, and Tn indicates the reference duration for that level as given in Table G-16a of the OSHA noise regulation. Doses greater than 100% exceed the OSHA PEL.

When noise exposures exceed the PEL of 90 dBA, OSHA requires that employees wear hearing protection and that an employer implement feasible engineering or administrative controls to reduce noise exposures. The OSHA noise standard also requires an employer to implement a hearing conservation program when 8-hour TWA noise exposures exceed the AL 85 dBA. The program must include noise monitoring, employee notification, observation, audiometric testing, hearing protectors, training, and record keeping.

NIOSH [NIOSH 1998] and ACGIH [ACGIH 2011] recommend an exposure limit of 85 dBA as an 8-hour TWA. A more conservative 3 dB exchange rate is used in calculating these exposure limits. Using NIOSH criteria, an employee can be exposed to 85 dBA for 8 hours, but to no more than 88 dBA for 4 hours, 91 dBA for 2 hours, 94 dBA for 1 hour, etc. According to the NIOSH REL, 12-hour exposures must be 83.2 dBA or less.

Audiometric evaluations of employees' hearing thresholds must be conducted in quiet locations, preferably in a sound-attenuating booth, by presenting pure tones of varying frequencies at threshold levels (i.e., the level of a sound that the person can just barely hear). Zero dB hearing level represents the hearing level of an average, young individual with good hearing. OSHA requires hearing thresholds to be measured at test frequencies of 500, 1,000, 2,000, 3,000, 4,000, and 6,000 Hz. Individual employee's annual audiograms are compared to their baseline audiogram to determine if a standard threshold shift has occurred. OSHA states that a standard threshold shift has occurred if the average threshold values at 2,000, 3,000, and 4,000 Hz have increased by 10 dB or more in either ear when comparing the annual audiogram to the baseline audiogram [29 CFR 1910.95]. The NIOSH-recommended hearing threshold shift criterion is a 15-dB shift at any frequency in either ear from 500–6,000 Hz measured twice in succession [NIOSH 1998]. Both of these hearing threshold shift criteria require at least two audiometric tests.

The audiogram profile is a plot of the hearing test frequencies (x-axis) versus the hearing threshold levels (y-axis). For many employees, the audiogram profile tends to slope downward toward the high frequencies with an improvement at the audiogram's highest frequencies, forming a "notch" [Suter 2002]. A notch in the audiogram of an employee with otherwise normal hearing may indicate the early onset of hearing loss. The notch from occupational noise can occur between 3,000 and 6,000 Hz [ACOM 1989; Osguthorpe and Klein 2001]. However, it is generally accepted that a notch at 4,000 Hz indicates occupational hearing loss [Prince et al. 1997]. An individual may have notches at different frequencies in one or both ears [Suter 2002]. For this evaluation, a notch is defined as the frequency where the hearing level is preceded by an improvement of at least 10 dB and followed by an improvement of at least 5 dB.

References

ACOM [1989]. Occupational noise-induced hearing loss. ACOM Noise and Hearing Conservation Committee. J Occup Med 31(12):996.

ACGIH [2011]. 2011 TLVs® and BEIs®: threshold limit values for chemical substances and physical agents and biological exposure indices. Cincinnati, OH: American Conference of Governmental Industrial Hygienists.

AIHA [2011]. AIHA 2011 Emergency response planning guidelines (ERPG) & workplace environmental exposure levels (WEEL) handbook. Fairfax, VA: American Industrial Hygiene Association.

Berger EH, Royster LH, Royster JD, Driscoll DP, Layne M, eds. [2003]. The noise manual. 5th rev. ed. Fairfax, VA: American Industrial Hygiene Association.

Brown-Williams H, Lichterman J, Kosnett M [2009]. Indecent exposure: lead puts workers and families at risk. Health Research in Action, University of California, Berkeley. Perspectives 4(1)1–9.

CDC [2005]. Preventing Lead Poisoning in Young Children. Atlanta: CDC; 2005. [http://www.cdc.gov/nceh/lead/publications/prevleadpoisoning.pdf]. Date accessed: September 2011.

CFR. Code of Federal Regulations. Washington, DC: U.S. Government Printing Office, Office of the Federal Register.

CSTE [2009]. Public health reporting and national notification for elevated blood lead levels. CSTE position statement 09-OH-02. Atlanta: CSTE 2009 [http://www.cste.org/ps2009/09-OH-02.pdf]. Date accessed: September 2011.

Farfel MR, Chisholm JJ [1990]. Health and environmental outcomes of traditional and modified practices for abatement of residential lead–based paint. Am J Pub Health 80(10):1240–1245.

Grandjean P, Bach E [1986]. Indirect exposures: the significance of bystanders at work and at home. Am Ind Hyg Assoc J 47(12):819–824.

Lauwerys RR, Hoet P [2001]. Chapter 2. Biological monitoring of exposure to inorganic and organometallic substances. In: Industrial chemical exposure: guidelines for biological monitoring. 3rd ed. Boca Raton, FL: CRC Press, LLC, pp. 21–180.

Moline JM, Landrigan PJ [2005]. Lead. Chapter 39.8. In: Textbook of clinical occupational and environmental medicine, Rosenstock L, Cullen MR, Brodkin CA, and Redlich CA, eds., 2nd ed. Philadelphia, PA: Elsevier Saunders, pp. 967–979.

NCEH [2005]. Third national report on human exposure to environmental chemicals. Atlanta, GA: U.S. Department of Health and Human Services, Centers for Disease Control and Prevention. National Center for Environmental Health Publication number 05–0570.

NIOSH [1998]. Criteria for a recommended standard: occupational noise exposure (revised criteria 1998). Cincinnati, OH: U.S. Department of Health and Human Services, Centers for Disease Control and Prevention, National Institute for Occupational Safety and Health, DHHS (NIOSH) Publication No. 98-126.

NIOSH [2010]. NIOSH pocket guide to chemical hazards. Cincinnati, OH: U.S. Department of Health and Human Services, Centers for Disease Control and Prevention, National Institute for Occupational Safety and Health, DHHS (NIOSH) Publication No. 2010-168c. [http://www.cdc.gov/niosh/npg/]. Date accessed: September 2011.

Osguthorpe JD, Klein AJ [2001]. Occupational hearing conservation. Clin Audiol 24(2):403–414.

Prince M, Stayner L, Smith R, Gilbert S [1997]. A re-examination of risk estimates from the NIOSH Occupational Noise and Hearing Survey (ONHS). J Acous Soc Am 101(2):950–963.

Schwartz BS, Hu H [2007]. Adult lead exposure: time for change. Environ Health Perspect 115(3):451–454.

Schwartz BS, Stewart WF [2007]. Lead and cognitive function in adults: A question and answers approach to a review of the evidence for cause, treatment, and prevention. Int Rev Psychiatry 19(6):671–692.

Sussell A [1998]. Protecting workers exposed to lead-based paint hazards: a report to congress. Cincinnati, OH: U.S. Department of Health and Human Services, Centers for Disease Control and Prevention, National Institute for Occupational Safety and Health, DHHS (NIOSH) Publication No. 98–112.

Suter AH [1978]. The ability of mildly hearing-impaired individuals to discriminate speech in noise. Washington, DC: U.S. Environmental Protection Agency, Joint EPA/USAF study, EPA 550/9-78-100, AMRL-TR-78-4.

Suter AH [2002]. Hearing conservation manual. 4th ed. Milwaukee, WI: Council for Accreditation in Occupational Hearing Conservation.

Appendix B: Methods

Noise Dosimetry

Noise dosimeters (Larson Davis, Provo, Utah, Spark™ models 706RC or 705P) were attached to the wearer's belt, and a small remote microphone was fastened to the wearer's shirt at a point midway between the ear and outside of the shoulder. A windscreen provided by the dosimeter manufacturer was placed over the microphone to reduce or eliminate artifact noise, which can occur if objects bump against an unprotected microphone. The dosimeters were set up to collect data using different settings to allow comparison of noise measurement results with the three different noise exposure limits referenced in this health hazard evaluation, the OSHA PEL and AL and the NIOSH REL (Table B1). During noise dosimetry measurements, noise levels below the threshold level are not integrated by the dosimeter for accumulation of dose and calculation of TWA noise level.

The dosimeters averaged noise levels every second. At the end of the sampling period, the dosimeter was removed and paused to stop data collection. The noise measurement information stored in the dosimeters was downloaded to a computer for interpretation with Larson Davis Blaze® software. The dosimeters were calibrated before and after the measurement periods according to the manufacturer's instructions.

Table B1. Dosimeter settings

Parameters	OSHA AL	OSHA PEL	NIOSH REL
Response	Slow	Slow	Slow
Exchange rate	5	5	3
Criterion level	90	90	85
Threshold	80	90	80
Upper limit	115	115	115

Area noise levels and octave band noise frequency analysis (measurement of noise in different frequencies) were measured with System 824 SLM and real-time frequency analyzers (Larson-Davis, Provo, Utah). The SLMs were equipped with 0.25-inch random incidence Type 1 microphones; the instruments measured noise levels between 16 and 170 dBA. Sound level and octave band frequency spectrum measurements were collected at a sample rate of 51,200 times per second and averaged eight times per second. The SLMs were calibrated before and after the measurement periods according to the manufacturer's instructions. SLMs were either handheld or mounted on a tripod at a height of approximately 5 feet.

Lead in Air

Air samples for lead were collected on 37-millimeter diameter, 0.8-micron pore-size mixed cellulose ester filters using SKC Air Check® 2000 air sampling pumps (SKC Inc., Eighty Four, Pennsylvania) calibrated at a flow rate of 2 liters per minute. The inlet port of the sampling pump was connected to the sampling media with Tygon® tubing. For PBZ samples, the sampling media were attached to the employee's lapel within the breathing zone, roughly defined as an area in front of the shoulders with a radius of 6 to 9 inches. Samples were analyzed by inductively coupled plasma according to NIOSH Method 7303 [NIOSH 2011].

Lead on Surfaces

We collected six surface wipe samples for lead. Surface samples were collected with premoistened Palintest® dust wipes (Palintest USA, Erlanger, Kentucky). The collection procedure was as follows: (1) identify the area to be sampled, (2) put on a pair of disposable nitrile gloves, (3) place the wipe flat on surface as defined by the 10 centimeter by 10 centimeter disposable template and wipe surface using three to four horizontal S-strokes, side-to-side so that entire surface is covered, (4) wipe the area with three to four vertical S-strokes, (5) wipe the area with three to four diagonal S-strokes, and (6) place the wipe in a sterile container. A new template and a pair of disposable gloves were used for each wipe sample. The wipe samples were digested and analyzed by inductively coupled argon plasma according to NIOSH Method 9102 [NIOSH 2011].

Lead on Hands

Hand wipe samples were collected and analyzed with a commercially available dust wipe (Full Disclosure® Instant Wipes, SKC Inc., Eighty Four, Pennsylvania) conforming to the American Society for Testing and Materials Standard E 1792 (Specifications for Wipe Sampling Materials for Lead in Surface Wipes). After collection, each wipe was sprayed with a 5% leaching solution of acetic acid to solubilize lead and lead compounds into lead ions. The wipe was then sprayed with a chilled solution of sodium rhodizonate, a chemical that reacts colorimetrically to the presence of lead by changing from yellow to red. The visual limit of identification for the method is approximately 17–20 micrograms per sample.

Reference

NIOSH [2011]. NIOSH manual of analytical methods (NMAM®), 4th ed. Schlecht PC, O'Connor PF, eds. Cincinnati, OH: U.S. Department of Health and Human Services, Centers for Disease Control and Prevention, National Institute for Occupational Safety and Health, DHHS (NIOSH) Publication 94–113 (August, 1994); 1st Supplement Publication 96–135, 2nd Supplement Publication 98–119; 3rd Supplement 2003–154. http://www.cdc.gov/niosh/nmam/. Date accessed: September 2011.

Acknowledgments and
Availability of Report

The Hazard Evaluations and Technical Assistance Branch (HETAB) of the National Institute for Occupational Safety and Health (NIOSH) conducts field investigations of possible health hazards in the workplace. These investigations are conducted under the authority of Section 20(a)(6) of the Occupational Safety and Health Act of 1970, 29 U.S.C. 669(a)(6) which authorizes the Secretary of Health and Human Services, following a written request from any employer or authorized representative of employees, to determine whether any substance normally found in the place of employment has potentially toxic effects in such concentrations as used or found. HETAB also provides, upon request, technical and consultative assistance to federal, state, and local agencies; labor; industry; and other groups or individuals to control occupational health hazards and to prevent related trauma and disease.

Mention of any company or product does not constitute endorsement by NIOSH. In addition, citations to websites external to NIOSH do not constitute NIOSH endorsement of the sponsoring organizations or their programs or products. Furthermore, NIOSH is not responsible for the content of these websites. All Web addresses referenced in this document were accessible as of the publication date.

This report was prepared by Lilia Chen and Scott E. Brueck of HETAB, Division of Surveillance, Hazard Evaluations and Field Studies. Health communication assistance was provided by Stefanie Evans. Editorial assistance was provided by Ellen Galloway. Desktop publishing was performed by Robin Smith and Greg Hartle.

Copies of this report have been sent to employee and management representatives, the state health department, and the Occupational Safety and Health Administration Regional Office. This report is not copyrighted and may be freely reproduced. The report may be viewed and printed at http://www.cdc.gov/niosh/hhe/. Copies may be purchased from the National Technical Information Service at 5825 Port Royal Road, Springfield, Virginia 22161.